# Roman Lee

# How to improve your eyesight and fulfill yourself as an individual.

## Table of contents

# Author's Preface.

You are holding the book, which is written for you in order to help you improve your eyesight, to awaken the abilities, which are hidden in your soul, and to fulfill yourself as an Individual.

This is the method of rapid visual recovery after an emotional volitional self-restraint. It is based on the Eastern teachings, scientific works and my experience as a pharmacist. I have already tested this method successfully.

There is a simple formula: THE CHARACTER AND DESTINY EQUAL DISEASE. Hence, in order to improve your health and life in general, you need to change the character.

This textbook is written for those who consider themselves to be outstanding PEOPLE in their lives and strive to improve or restore the eyesight through their own efforts and hard work.

You have to warm to the role of the creative INDIVIDUAL.

Nature abhors a vacuum. Any work gives some result, but it only depends on you how big it will be! There isn't anything which can exist from nothing, from the void.

When you inspire respect through the efforts of your will, increase your self-esteem artificially, deepen faith in your power, all this will be reflected in every cell of the body and on your behavior, actions and deeds.

Due to the repetition of the action habit is created, there is character formation, and fate is created. There is little bigger self-esteem today than yesterday and tomorrow it will make you a little bit different. Hence, you will gradually become the person who you are going to be, and you will overcome all the life's difficulties with a passion for sport.

# About the system.

This method defies not the disease but the patient with chronic disease! Not a disease is a killer but a chronically ill, who doesn't want to change anything in himself. Most people are lazy. It is easier to see the world through an intermediary, that is, through the glasses rather than to be busy with books, especially to learn something through them. It is impossible to change human nature from the outside. It is melted from the inside, by the man himself, by his desire, aspiration and his iron will. The system is designed for strong people, because it implies active participation.

No technique can change a person's soul. And if a sick person is passive and is waiting for "recovering his health" through droplets, procedures, special glasses, he is doomed to eternal waiting, because he hopes that the next time he "will be given" again. And then it will be much harder for him to "get" it because safety margin of the organism is depleted by disease: it reduces and becomes smaller and smaller.

The patient hopes and does nothing. But if he puts his hands to it by his own efforts, he stands shoulder to shoulder with his doctor against this disease, then victory is assured.

Opportunities of the organism aren't limited.

# The plan of work.

First. Get acquainted with laziness and with many hidden forms of its essence.

Second. Explore the art of creation.

Third. Insure against all kinds of errors towards the goal.

Fourth. Put locomotor apparatus in order, strengthen the muscles in order to organize the functioning of internal organs, conduct vision correction.

Fifth. Deal with your experiences, problems and aspirations.

You can retort: why should I train my back, if I have myopia? But the eyes aren't isolated from other organs and everything is interconnected.

Our goal is to eliminate the cause of the disease. If we remove the cause, the consequences will disappear.

That is why this rehabilitation system is so effective.

Mastering this system, you will not only improve your health, but also will be able to fulfill yourself as an individual, be creative, find job which is right for you and become rich, and not only spiritually. But you will achieve this only under one condition – by knowing yourself.

By knowing yourself you know God!

There is nothing fantastic, this is reality.

But the main secret underlying this system is a way of behavior of the patient, his attitude to himself and his life.

If you add this attitude to the treatment, which is prescribed you by doctor, you can overcome together almost any disease.

When a patient believes and hopes that he will be cured by someone, the doctor remains alone with his illness. It holds one of the secrets of chronic failures in all spheres of life.

For decades, the patient tries to recover by approaching logically to solving health problems. He says: "At first, give me health, and then I will believe in the outcome and rejoice."

From the viewpoint of the normal person, he does the things right, that is, he rejoices only after he sees the outcome. It is logical!

The effect is obtained, faith appears, then mood improves and, of course, "muscular corset" (posture and gestures) are like the winners have. A face becomes satisfied and your smile shines. Here is a scheme of a typical behavior of unhappy person:

I doubt, don't believe, hope etc. Give me the positive outcome

Then I will believe

**Then I will be in a good mood**


And I will hold the "muscle corset", which is inherent to a happy person.


Since I don't believe, my body isn't mobilized, since it isn't mobilized, I won't recover, and I will have even more convincing argument for unbelief. That is the logic of death; the logic of suicide and the logic of the unfortunate loser.

# Where is the way out of this situation?

Are you ready to turn everything upside down? Then we carry out in practice absolutely illogical approach to logical being stuck in the disease.

First we take "muscular corset", that is, we straighten our back, straighten our shoulders and we grin from ear to ear. In other words, we deliberately create a posture and gestures of the WINNER.

Then we evoke inner state of joy artificially.

Then we form a mental image of recovery, we force ourselves to believe in the success of the recovery by the effort of will.

If you behave like this, the result will be always with you, without even asking your permission!

Look at the approximate formula of action of the human, who is doomed to succeed in life:

Willful compulsion

"Muscle corset"

Mood

## Faith

## Outcome!

If the "muscular corset" changes, then emotions and thoughts have to be changed too, since their synchronization with the emotional center occurs.

Here we come to the essence of action of the mechanism. There is a center of the synchronization of muscles, mood and thoughts. Simply put, emotions are transmitted to the brain through our blood and they affect the condition of our organisms.

Now the tricky question is: What is easier to do: to lift the mood, change your thoughts or to keep the muscles in a certain position? The mood is volatile, it can be hold for a few seconds, then you are a little distracted - and the mood changes immediately.

**Conditioned reflex.** This reflex is acquired by the action of indifferent stimulus. Another way of occurrence of reflex is habit formation, which is formed by repetition. Recovery occurs due to the elimination of "reflex of poor eyesight."

# Mistakes.

## Lack of the objective.

If we don't know what goal we have to achieve, then how can we define that we have already achieved it?

The second thing. The patient recovers when he has a goal, an internal aspiration or craving for recovery.

**If the person directs attention to an unhealthy organ every day, gets into positive mood, tracks the results, then the recovery mechanism is launched.**

After doing exercises, don't forget to thank the body sincerely, and to create a physically tangible sense of gratitude inside you.

No matter what medicine you will give him, no matter what exercises you will do with him, if he doesn't set a well-defined task and doesn't work on every unhealthy section of his body every day, the recovery will be greatly delayed or won't occur at all.

The move without a goal is a "way you don't know where it goes". But the implementation of the task should be kept under strict control...

## Laziness.

The most direct and sincere form of it is this expression: "I don't want! I won't!"

Do you remember? The boundary between health and illness is faith. If your answer is on the other side of the "barricades", then you are simply lazy! You are hiding behind the explanations and arguments in order not to work on yourself.

Let us analyze for clarity what a doubt is.

Figuratively speaking, a doubt is the eyes which are located at the back of the head. They can only look back at the past, at the experienced failures and defeats. And any move forward is accompanied with new dashes against the rock. And the farther you go, the more teeth you cut.

The negative experience continues to accumulate and to strengthen in your mind. Hence, the uncertainty in your power increases. You peer into yesterday more vigilantly, convincing yourself and others that there is no future without the past.

It turns out that chronic failures are an implemented doubt. A doubt is an aggressive form of laziness.

Only laziness, driving into the framework of generally accepted concepts, thinking, behavior, actions, makes you live, think and act like everyone else, it ultimately leads to a deadlock. Separate yourself from the crowd! Get out of this swamp!

An outstanding, brilliant, strong personality lies in everyone but, unfortunately, it isn't discovered. You have to give the opportunity to your true deep essence of HUMAN to be expressed. Sitting on a gold mountain, you go begging, being neck-deep in spring water, and you are dying of thirst! This is a sacrilege!

Knowing ourselves, we know God! This means that everything is put in us by the Lord God: our will to love and create. We have to admit and develop it, and we will go on in order to achieve it.

The most common mistake and the greatest danger lie in self-dissatisfaction.

Low self-esteem is the most terrible and destructive power, it is a kind of death. Hatred is poison. The man, who hates himself, hates others.

A person, who does not respect himself, will not be able to respect the other.

A person, who does not love himself and does not accept who he is, is unable to love.

You will not be able to give what you don't have. In one of the holy books the Lord God says: "Love your neighbor as yourself."

Now we are discussing the most destructive sides of nature of the chronically ill loser. But character can be changed for the better by making the efforts of will.

So, the first task is to write down all the negative traits, which you want to remove, in a column, and near the negative traits you have to write down all the positive traits that you would like to strengthen and develop. This task is the foundation for many exercises, which will be discussed below.

When you believe that you are a great INDIVIDUAL, when you know that you are the most beautiful woman in the world, that you are a cool man, then the appearance and behavior, and the results of all your efforts will meet the internal state. Thoughts are material. Self-reliance will be reflected everywhere, in your body and in every cell!

The ancients said: "Think before you think".

And you have to remember that love, self-respect and any attention to yourself can't be lost without a trace.

# Accident prevention.

1. From the first days of doing exercises don't draw negative conclusions about yourself and your abilities.

2. Always work on your eyesight, even with your eyes closed, without glasses!

3. Get the glasses which are weaker than those that you normally wear and put them on today. With the improvement of your eyesight, these glasses will be "large" for you too.

Change them as long as the demand for glasses doesn't disappear.

If you go on wearing your old glasses, then don't even dream about success!
In the early days of the work with the eye chart the improvement will be barely noticeable, gently, at a slow pace. And all, which have been achieved recently, will be very unsteady.

If you wear old glasses for at least 5 minutes, a long-standing habit of wearing "bike" on the nose for decades will immediately instantly be recalled. And then it will be much harder to go back to the accumulated result.

Building is more difficult than breaking! The work, with the help of which you will reach your goal, is easy to be destroyed. You have to close the way back in your soul, only then you will advance.

4. If you can do it without glasses, it refers to those who have vision 1.5-2 dpt., then you should say goodbye to them

today. Don't wear them anywhere else. The glasses are a pair of crutches for the eyes.

5. During vision correction, don't screw up your eyes and goggle. You should work without overstrain.

6. Don't hurry! Your plan is one line of the eye chart for two or three days, 0.25 dpt. per day.

Then rest from 1 to 2 days!

7. There is no room for complacency, just go on working! Once you calm down, stop, relax, eyesight will cease to improve. Do you remember? Flywheel - inertia - stop.

# «Meditation». What is it?

This is the name of special exercise, which is aimed at the awakening of the latent power, that everyone has from the nature, and that will lead you to recovery.

What is the "Meditation"?

This is a particular exercise for training your Spirit! Now I will try to explain you what feelings and sensations you have to induce.

Imagine you return home after a long absence, but at home you find your child waiting for you. You are happy, shivers run up and down your spine, when you imagine that you will take him in your arms, he will embrace you with his little hands, cuddle, will kiss you with his plump, moist lips. You will feel the breath of your child and everything will cease to exist for you!

You will feel that you are strong, powerful patron, titanium and defender. The soul will be filled with purity, tenderness, bliss and love due to this!

These feelings and experiences are the foundation and the internal support for your best aspirations, on which your goal will be built.

And at the same time "Meditation" is the driving force for the implementation of your objective.

"Meditation" is an art of controlling your body, ordering it to do something and forcing it to gradually transform externally and internally into THAT form which you want.

This statement, this internal feeling is that it will be as you want it!!

"Meditation" is a conscious creation of confidence and power in your soul!

"Meditation" is a combination of confidence, determination, strength, power, hardness and tenderness, love, kindness, trepidation, an illusion of flying and joy.

This condescending tranquility and quiet confident knowledge that everything will be as you want it!

Your "Meditation" should tear all the uncertainties, doubts and fears to shreds. Destroy them all!

Try to feel your importance, strength, power, beauty, try to approve it in yourself and move toward your goal step by step.

Try to piece out this feeling with new shades, with new range of feelings every day. As you train, you will become calmer, stronger, more confident person, the protection, encouragement and support for the people who surround you. You will become an oasis in the desert for them; you will bring light, goodness and love.

When you start working with the eyes, you will direct the feeling, the statement, and the command to the eyes to be what you want them to be. You create joy there and get feedback.

It may be warmth, light pulsation, or any other physical response. "Meditation" is internal merger with the image of youthfulness, which have just been created by you.

But, as always, you have to observe regulations for ensuring safety. Make sure that the heart is working quietly, your head is clear, and breath sounds are equal. Inside you there is condescending tranquility and absolute knowledge of that fact that everything will be as you want it.

You should know that any of your problems can be solved easily, that you are the best in all respects.

No stress! In other words, your task is to keep your body under control, and recovery will take place as if by itself. This should be the tranquility of master, creator, peace loving, loved and powerful man. Create this affirmation!

The inner aspiration has to be very strong. This inner affirmation is like that:

I AM WILL
I AM STRENGHTH
I AM LOVE
I AM FORGIVENESS
I AM POWER
I AM JUVENESENCE
I AM YOUTHFULNESS
I AM HEALTH
I AM WISDOM
I AM BUOYANCY
I AM EVERYTHING WONDERFUL
ALL DEPENDS ON ME
EVERYTHING IN MY HANDS

This aspiration should dominate and destroy all doubts, which will not go away by itself.

This exercise is always applied during vision correction or working with any other unhealthy body, during articular gymnastics and eye exercises, as well as during erasing the laundry, cleaning the apartment, shaking in the public transport and so on. D. And especially after the unpleasant conversation with the head or in other vital moments.

This exercise should be done on the street, among the people.

Very important note! When you do the exercises, and your head is full of extraneous thoughts, all your efforts will be a waste of time!

The entire work will go down the drain during the mechanical performance. It is necessary to do in the condition of "Meditation"! Only then you will achieve success!

Every morning you have to force yourself to feel that you are:

tranquility,
heartfulness,
buoyancy,
tenderness,
beauty,
fascination,
kindness,
strenghth,
love,
power!

Just do it!

"Meditation" is the foundation upon which all of your Creation is held on.

During the "Meditation" you are giving the order. You are building yourself, it all depends on you! Pay attention to it!

The spirit is the winner!

Now with the help of "Meditation" we proceed to exercise the Spirit! So, "Meditation" is not only recognition of you as an INDIVIDUAL and THE CREATOR.

This is a TRANSFORMATION into kind, strong, gentle man, a man who knows how to forgive, who has the ability to appreciate people and all their advantages and disadvantages. This is an internal ORDER of health, strength, beauty, kindness, light, love, happiness...

Try to create an internal impulse, inner aspiration for healing and feeling a sense of excitement for the fact that you are working on yourself, that you are recovering!

We all have a lot of doubts and disbelief. Where will a ten-year experience of being unhealthy vanish? They won't disappear by themselves! They need to be torn to shreds by the self-respect and faith in your strength!

"Meditation" is the complete opposite of doubt and disbelief; it is an active creation!

# Eye chart.

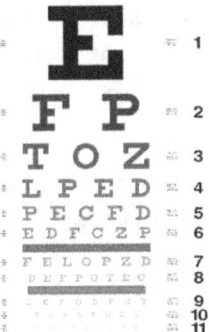

Eye chart for vision correction is an indicator of the correctness of your work with emotions, that is, it is necessary for controlling your emotions. You can buy or print IT.

By itself, the table does not give you anything because it's just a piece of paper. Do not expect that there will be a miracle, create it by yourself!

Your task is to direct 90% of your efforts to "muscle corset" and your mood. That's all!

You have to hold your "muscle corset" and lift up your mood as long as you don't take hold of your eyesight.

The table will show whether you work or just look at it, expecting that there is something to see.

If you don't work hard inside of you, you don't create the right mood, then you can wait for improvement for at least a hundred years, you won't get it! So, in other words, this sheet of paper is an indicator of your character. If the character is lousy, then...

But when you recognize yourself as a great MAN, a strong and confident INDIVIDUAL, your eyesight will begin to obey you, and the result will grow like an avalanche.

So, when you pick up an eye chart, first of all, you have to check your posture and gestures. And look at it as if in passing. Don't try to look at it through your eyes.

## How to hold the table and how to work in every particular case?

1. If you have hyperopia (that is, you wear glasses for near vision), keep an eye chart in front of the eyes at a distance of 15-20 cm.

2. If you have myopia (that is, you wear glasses for distance), you have to keep it at arm's length. If you have low myopia, when you see well the last line in the table at a distance, hang it on the wall and find the row for you. Read below how to do it.

3. People who see badly both near and far, that is, who have astigmatism, can work as well as they have myopia or hyperopia, there is no difference, because your result doesn't depend on it.

4. One eye sees normally, but the other sees badly. Make an eye bandage for a healthy eye or cover it with your hand. Hold an eye chart at distance for you according to the diopters.

5. Both eyes see badly, but one sees even worse. You have to work on both eyes. One of them will recover faster, and then proceed as in the previous case.

6. One eye is farsighted and the other is nearsighted. Since we will work with this eye chart twice a day, then once a

day we will work on one eye (the other is covered by an eye bandage), similarly, once a day we will work on the other eye.

7. If you have glaucoma, cataracts, optic atrophy, retinal degeneration. You have to work under the general scheme, but you have to pay special attention to eye relaxation exercises. I warn you that you will move a little slower than the rest. It's alright! It all depends on your mood and aspiration.

## How to find the row for you in an eye chart?

You start to look at an eye chart with the top row, and gradually lowering the gaze, you will find the one above which you can see well, below which everything is fading away, that is, you have to find the border row. This is a row for you.

Once it will be clearly visible for you, you move the border below.

Attention!

Don't hurry to move the border, even if your eyes will "require" it. Entrench your results!

During working with an eye chart, there is often a passion, which is inappropriate in this case. Restrain it if you don't want to stall the process of restoring your eyesight!!!

This is accident prevention. Slow and steady wins the race.

If, working on myopia, you will clearly see the last row at arm's length, hang an eye chart on the wall and then reselect the row for work in the manner described above.

You know that the eyes are a part of the brain. They are indirectly connected with all organs. A person perceives about 80% of the information through his eyes, and only about 20% - through other sense organs.

Our eyes reflect our health, state of mind and mood.

You can see whether a person is good or bad, sick or healthy through his eyes. It isn't said in vain: "The eyes are the mirror of the soul".

They "respond" very quickly to the attention from your side, so, when you start to work with them, you will improve your eyesight quickly.

It is not so evident with other organs, and so, by force of habit, we are often mistaken, and we continue to mourn, throwing mud at ourselves: "I can't do it, I'm not like the others", etcetera.

And when you immediately receive dividends from your work, you will not have the right to doubt your abilities!

So, we apply the formula.

We form "muscle corset" by an effort of will, that is, posture and gestures of a healthy, happy, prancing man, of a young stallion, if you are a man, and of a happy mare, if you are a woman.

# Relaxation Exercises.

**1. Open your eyes slowly and quietly! Blink easy, without stress, like a butterfly with its wings.**

**2. And now the exercise called "Relax"**

**Firstly, turn on some pleasant and relaxing music.**

**Warm your palms in order to strengthen the flow of energy to them. Put your arms down to the level of the solar plexus, the energy will flow better if you do this. Going on rubbing, you will have to bring your hands to your eyes.**

**Put one hand on the other, fingers are tightly connected and crossed on the forehead and the base of the little fingers, which are connected at one point, are placed strictly on the bridge, in the place on which there is an earpiece. Make a cup with your palms.**

**Put them so that the light doesn't penetrate inside, and don't let your eyelashes touch the palms at the same time. Only then you have to close your eyes with your eyelids.**

**The energy from the center of the palms will go straight to the eyeballs. Your head should be in one plane with the spine so that the energy can come smoothly.**

**"Release" your eyeballs back, let your eyelids and face relax. Jaws are decompressed, the mouth isn't pressed down, shoulders are slumped, and hands are without strain. The muscles of the whole body are relaxed.**

Please, create the state of renunciation, tranquility, thoughtlessness and emptiness. We observe the darkness or any image that arises in our mind.

You can observe the moving objects mentally, and at such a distance, where you can see physically ill, and on an imaginary level it is very clear even at this distance. You can imagine an object at close distance, then at the far distance.

During relaxation it is very useful to observe mentally your row of work in an eye chart and to imagine that you see it clearly and accurately!

Exercise "Guiding of energy to the eyes".

Firstly, we have to rub the palms, as it is described in the exercise called "Relax".

The body is straight; head is aligned with the spine. Eyes are closed. The index and middle fingers of both hands are directed perpendicularly to the eyes.

The distance from the fingertips to the eye literally is from 1 to 2 mm, but we don't touch the eyelids with our fingers. You have to feel how the energy flows in the eyes and fills them from the inside.

Now, the middle phalanges of thumbs (you need to bend your fingers for this) are brought to the closed eyelids, you have to fill your eyes with energy. The elbows are raised. You don't have to tilt your head.

# Eye exercises.

In the East there is an ancient method of diagnosing diseases by the move of an eye, not by the iris, but namely by the move of the eyeballs.

For example, specialist asks you to "draw" a circle with your eyes and looks how you're doing it.

It turns out, depending on the disease, that the eyes start to "cut" the corners somewhere, the line is uneven. This confirms once again that everything in our body is interconnected and interdependent.

But even the man can't follow the correct move of an eye, so you have to ask someone from your relatives to help you.

Doing exercises for the eyes correctly, we not only train the muscles, but also we work indirectly with unhealthy organs.

So, you have to follow this interesting process that the moves of your eyes have to clearly "draw" these lines during doing of exercises. Getting started!

How do you start any work on yourself? Do you remember?

Come on, straighten your shoulders. Firstly, hold "muscle corset". What do you need for this? Yeah, you are correct! You have to straighten your back and grin from ear to ear. Then, you have to induce positive emotions artificially inside yourself. How can you do it? You know this! Have you done it?

And now you can start to do the exercises. Just don't forget to blink!

1. Keep your head straight, don't throw it back. The sight is directed upwards (to the ceiling), and mentally you keep moving your eyes from the skull to top of your head, as if you are looking there.

2. And now drop your eyes down, and turn your attention to the thyroid gland, as if you are looking at that place where your throat is.

3. Look to the left: the eyes are looking at the wall, but the attention is on the left ear.

4. Look to the right: the eyes are looking at another wall, and the attention is on the right ear.

Why is it important to keep your eyes moving on the mental level during doing these well-known exercises?

It was known even in ancient times in the East that in the area of the crown there was a huge bundle of energy channels, and at the outer edge of the eye there was a center associated with bile ducts.

Therefore, going on moving of the eye mentally to the ear, thus, we affect the bile ducts and liver. The eyes are a window of the liver. I don't casually talk about it.

Behind the outward simplicity of all exercises for eyesight recovery the deeper meaning, which is rooted in antiquity, lies.

But, as in everything, there you also need to remember about the accident prevention. Don't overdo it. Any overstrain in the eye leads to the opposite result.

That's why here I want to draw your attention again to aforementioned eye relaxation exercises, which affect the entire organism beneficially.

5. "Butterfly". An indispensable condition for the exercise: head is static, you are working only on eyes. The "Picture" should be of the maximum possible size within your face, but the muscles of your eyeballs shouldn't be overstrained, observe your state!

Your sight should be shifted in the following order: to the lower left corner, to the upper right corner, to the lower right corner, to the upper left corner.

Now, vice versa: to the lower right corner, to the upper left corner, to the lower left corner, to the upper right corner. Now you have to relax, to blink frequently and easily, as a butterfly waving its wings. Never squint, never open your eyes very widely! Everything creates tension that is contraindicated!

6. "Eight". An indispensable condition for this exercise is the same as in the "Butterfly".

And now describe smoothly with your eyes a horizontal eight or the infinity symbol of maximum size within the face. You have to do it several times to the one side and then several times to the other side. You have to blink frequently and easily.

7. Exercises for people with strabismus.

Here oblique muscles of eye are operating. It is very effective when you have the nearsightedness. It promotes the development of peripheral vision.

Special note: this exercise should be done in a calm atmosphere. Nobody and nothing should scare you.

Look at your tip of the nose, squinting, or put a finger in front of you and look at it without being interrupted, gradually approaching it to the tip of the nose. Eyes converge.

Then look forward calmly and absently, and attention is spread around. That is, you have to check any items with peripheral vision, without taking a look at it!

And so alternately:

at the tip of the nose - forward and, without shifting a gaze, to the sides.

at the nose - forward and to the sides,

at the point between the eyebrows, and then again forward and, without shifting a gaze,  to the sides.

Go on doing this exercise for 7-8 times in each direction.

We shift our gaze from the point to the point smoothly and quietly.

Do the exercises slowly, feeling joy and gratitude to yourself. Is there a smile on your face? This is excellent! Check your internal state! Blink again and flutter your eyelashes.

8. Exercise for turning the axes of eyesight. Forefingers are brought to the tip of the nose and our eyes are looking at the forefingers. Then we start to turn our eyes to the different sides, slowly distancing our fingers from nose. The right eye follows

the right finger, and the left eye follows the left finger. I will give you a small prompt: it can be done only with peripheral vision.

Don't break your eyes! The goal is quite different! Then you have to repeat this exercise, squinting at the bridge. Don't forget to rest!

### 9. *"Big circle"*.

Do the circular motions with your eyeballs. The head remains static. Imagine a large gold-colored dial in front of you. This color helps restore vision.

Move your eyes slowly, noting each digit on an imaginary dial. At first, to one side, and then to the other.

Attention! You don't have to cut corners! Make sure that the line is straight. The radius of the circle will gradually increase.

You have to blink calmly; don't overstrain your eyes.

And now the same exercise, but your face is turned to the sky. Your eyes are opened.

Repeat this exercise in two versions in both directions, but with your eyes which are closed. At this time the crystalline lens is massaged.

There is joy in your soul because of the fact that you will see well, when you open your eyes. Create a reverent expectation of the result and at the same time the state of indulgent tranquility that it will be exactly what you want.

The exercises from 1 to 8 are done in three stages: at first, with your eyes open, then with your eyes closed, and then this exercise is repeated only mentally. At this time, there is an inner work at the cellular level.

I am drawing your attention particularly to the fact that the warm-up exercise for the eyes should be done in the order in which they are described, according to the degree of increasing of the complexity.

Remember!

Much tension on the eye leads to vision loss. Therefore, make sure of this tension, according to your feelings, and practice relaxation exercises more often (the more often - the better!).

# The massage of auricles.

Each move here and below should be made more than 8-10 times, first in one direction and then in the other.

The description will contain generic wordings such as "a few times" or simply "at first, in one direction and then in another direction"

This is done deliberately so that a mechanical counting of the number of repetitions won't preoccupy you.

The main thing is where you want to send your thoughts and mental strength. You know that all this should be sent for the internal state, for the formation of the positive aspects of your character which, from your point of view, aren't developed enough. In no case you don't have to incline to automatism. This is a road to nowhere.

There are more than thousands of biologically active points on the surface of your auricles, so, massaging them, we have an impact on the whole body indirectly. The mood I Take your ears, seize your auricles

Exercise 1.

Drag your ears down so that the inner ear is pulled back. In every move you have to put joy!

We have to alternate easy relaxation with more severe stress.

Then, similarly, you have to drag your ears up several times. I only ask you to observe the accident prevention! Don't tear off your ears!!!

Exercise 2.

Hold the middle of your auricle now. Grab it to the different sides and slightly back from the external auditory meatus. Grab your ears as far as possible with each new move, farther and farther...

If there is a feeling of stretching inside your ear, it means that you're doing it right. Well, how is it going? Are your ears there? This is excellent!

Exercise 3.

Now you have to do circular movements. Grab again your ear completely, hold in your hand as meat pasty.

You have to twist your ears. Are your ears burning?! This is very good! Shoulders should be straight! Take joy and pride in your work on yourself artificially. Your attention to yourself always materializes.

Exercise 4.

Change the clinch of your auricle. The palm is pressed to the ears by the base of the thumb so that there is a feeling of vacuum. (Palms are easy to be turned so that fingers are directed back.)

Make circular movements in both directions.

During the exercise, you have to create a feeling that you are powerful and all your commands are enforceable. Do you remember the exercise called "Meditation"?

Don't forget about your mood!!! You have to create the feeling that you are a strong person. Hold the internal image!

Exercise 5.

Be careful! This exercise must not be done by those who have a damaged eardrum or who don't have an eardrum at all!

Then we stop doing these movements. We press our hands to our ears firmly and tear our hands off sharply, so that there is a clap in our ear. We draw all the attention to our ears.

# Back strengthening exercises (articular gymnastics).

Many of the diseases of the internal organs are associated with the condition of the spine.

The spine is composed of interconnected vertebras. Between them there are cartilaginous intervertebral discs.

Vertebras execute the support function, and the disks are the absorbers of axial load and they give flexibility and mobility to the spine.

We are working with each part of the spine consistently:

with cervical spine,

with upper thoracic spine,

with lower thoracic spine,

with lumbar spine.

Before starting the exercises for the spine, you have to take deep inhalation through your nose and slow exhalation through your mouth. If you eat garlic or take a good drink, then you can do breathing exercises in front of mother-in-law.

Duration of an exhalation should be at least 3.2 times longer than an inhalation.

You absorb a physically perceived sense of youth, freshness and beauty with each breath. You have to create an image of strength, self-confidence, a sense of that fact that you can make your dream come true artificially by your own efforts.

Imagine that your eyes are healthy and they can clearly see even barely visible contours. Create an internal state of the victory over the disease artificially. Look at the disease from one side, and show the disease the door quietly, but very firmly and vigorously.

The most important is not just to instill it in yourself as a positive statement, but to create the inner feelings, which correspond to your thoughts, in the body artificially.

## The cervical spine.

Cervical spine training normalizes intracranial pressure, improves your eyesight, hearing, memory and increases your working ability.

Eventually, the vestibular apparatus restores, the state of the thyroid gland improves, sleeping becomes normal, numbness in hands is eliminated and brain power improves generally.

Exercise 1.

The body is straight; your chin is put down to your chest. Glide down the sternum with your chin, trying to reach the navel. When you reach the navel, you can go back!

Stress alternates with easy relaxation. We try to continue the movement with new stress, adding a little effort, and you have slight relaxation again. We make several movements.

But do it without feeling pain! The neck should feel pleasant straining. You have to create a wave of confidence in your abilities in the body artificially and try to keep it as long as possible.

Attention!
If you do this exercise very hard or if you have problems, which are connected with the cervical spine, you have to change these movements with your head and neck stretching forward.

### Exercise 2.

The body is straight, don't throw back your head, but lean it back slightly, the chin is pointed to the ceiling. Drag your chin up. Then, you have to stop the movements for a moment, but don't relax and drag your chin up again.

Make several of these movements, remembering about accident prevention.

### Exercise 3.

The spine is constantly straight. The shoulders are absolutely static during doing the exercises.

You have to tilt your head to the right (do not turn it!) and without much effort try to touch the shoulder with your ear.

Don't feel embarrassed if you don't reach the goal immediately. And do not overdo it! With the lapse of time, you will do it freely.

Then tilt your head to the left shoulder.

What trait are you working on now? Don't miss the opportunity to receive several awards for one work.

### Exercise 4.

You have to stand up straight. Head is straight, and you have to look ahead. Around the nose begin to turn the head to the right around the nose, as around the fixed pillar. Thus, chin is shifted to the right, slightly forward and upward.

Remember how a little puppy does it when he sees something interesting or responds to your words.

This exercise is done in three variants: the head is straight (look ahead), head is down (look at the floor), head is slightly tilted back (look at the ceiling). Be careful!

Exercise 5.

The circular movements of your head combine all the previous exercises into one exercise for the cervical spine.

The head rolls slowly and freely, without overstraining the muscles of the neck, several times in one direction and then several times in the other. Do it with the utmost care and attention. Keep track of your feelings.

If you have problems with the cervical spine, the movement is made on such a scheme: we are dragging the ear to the right shoulder, chin points down, then head slowly rolls to the left shoulder and back. That is, you have to do a part of a circle with your head, but don't tilt it back.

Exercise 6.

The body is straight. Stand up straight. Head is aligned to the spine.

Slowly we shift a gaze to the right, then we turn to the head. This is a starting position.

Trying to see what is behind your back, each time try to increase the angle of rotation by additional efforts. Don't throw your head back! Check it! Chin is near the shoulder!

Make several of these movements in one direction, then the same exercise to the other side. Overstrain is unacceptable! Don't forget to breathe!

Working with the upper thoracic and lower thoracic spine improves the cardiovascular and respiratory systems, removes the pain of intercostal neuralgia, improves the condition of the abdominal organs, kidneys, pancreas, and also eliminates numbness in your feet.

## The upper thoracic spine.

Exercise 1.

Stand up straight. The back is straight (no tilts!). The loin is static.

Arms are straight; they are linked to the lock below. Chin is pressed to your chest.

Shoulders are toward each other. We drag the chin to the navel, without riving it from the chest. Don't hold your breath!

The upper part of the spine takes the shape of an arc. Imagine that you have become to look like the hedgehog, which carries food stocks on the back. Repeat this movement several times. The amplitude is small.

Exercise 2.

You have to do the exercise similarly to the previous in the opposite direction.

We pull down straightened hands, which are clasped behind. Don't raise your shoulders! We keep our head straight and don't throw it back!

We bend the upper part of the spine in this position, chest takes a form of wheel (we strive upwards with our sternum).

Be careful. Don't overdo it!

Exercise 3.

The spine is straight. The loin is static. Your elbows are bent. We raise one shoulder, we bring the other shoulder down (as scales with different loading), and head tilts to the side of the shoulder, which is going down. We feel pleasant stress and tension in the upper thoracic spine.

Without changing position, you have to alternate stress with a slight relaxation, and each time we try to bend the spine a little more. No tilts! Keep an eye on it.

We do the same in the other direction. Don't hold your breath!

Exercise 4.

Spine is straight, we lean the pelvis or coccyx forward and fix it in this position.

Head is static, arms are by your side.

Bringing the shoulders down, we try to touch the floor with our arms. We feel the tension in the upper thoracic spine, and with each repetition we add a little effort after slight relaxation.

Imagine that a heavy bag is put on your shoulders. The spine becomes like a compressed spring under its weight. Hold this weight, add some effort, and help yourself with the movement of your shoulder downwards.

Look at your entire spine from top to bottom mentally and distribute this weight evenly.

Make sure that the load is not excessive.

Now we take this bag off. There is a feeling of lightness and flight.

You have to raise your shoulders against the stop, try to touch the ceiling with your top, the spine is stretched.

We alternate this movement of raising your shoulders with easy relaxation several times.

Imagine how all the vertebrae are straightened up and they slip back into place.

What about your thoughts in your head, huh? Do you remember? Everything develops with training! And it develops not only in body but also in your soul.

Exercise 5.

We have to make circular motions with our shoulders, combining it with the previous exercises. At first, the shoulder joints are rotated forward. Then we do the same thing in the opposite direction.

The upper part of the spine works actively.

Exercise 6.

Attention! The spine is the axis of rotation.

Your feet are "glued" to the floor and they are parallel to each other (toes are slightly directed inward), hands are on the shoulders, and you are looking ahead. Turn our eyes, head, shoulders and chest successively. Your abdomen, hips and legs are static.

The right arm goes to the right and pulls the left arm. If the abdomen and hips follow the movement of the right, this is a mistake. Try to return them original position, not changing position.

The tension arises in the shoulder girdle and in upper thoracic spine. You try to turn yourself even further.

We make a few springy movements with minimum amplitude, that is, we create additional stress and relaxation each time. We aim to increase the angle of rotation due to the new efforts.

Attention! We are strained at a slow exhalation!

Similarly, we do the exercises to the left. Have you learnt the technical side of this exercise? This is excellent!

## Lower thoracic spine.

Exercise 1.

We have to work in the same way as in the exercise № 1 for the upper thoracic spine. But we work on the spine from the neck to the waist.

The coccyx is leaned forward and we have to fix this position, that is, the pelvis is static.

As if we enfold something big and round with our hands.

A head is tilted down.

The spine is curved like an arch from the base of the skull to loins.

Add some tension. Reduce and add some tension again. No tilts!
In this position, you have to move your hands and to feel the muscles are playing and rolling back.
Exercise 2.

And now make the movements, which are reversed the previous movements. Don't throw your head back. Hands are up and laid back. Bring together your shoulder blades. Don't bend your loins!

Exercise 3.

Bend the right hand behind your head, elbow is directed to the ceiling, and look at the ceiling. Left shoulder is directed down.

We stretch our right side, alternating tension with a slight relaxation. The amplitude of the oscillations is small. Spine takes the form of an arc. No tilts! Change your hand. Do the same thing to the right several times.

Exercise 4.

Not only shoulders are involved in these movements, but also your head and the entire spine to the tailbone. You have to learn this exercise.

We stand up straight; feet are wider than shoulders, knees are slightly bent.

Head is straight, you have to look ahead and raise your shoulders to the ears.

We tilt our head down and shoulders aim to meet each other. Spine takes the form of an arc. Be careful, this is not the tilt!

Shoulders are coming down gradually, head is aligned.

Shoulders are moving back, your head is tilting back carefully, the spine is tilting forward.

And now we have to combine all these movements into one movement and to distribute the weight across the spine to the tailbone.

You have to remember visually how the wheels of a steam locomotive are spinning?

Do this exercise forward several times, and then you have to do it similarly in the opposite direction (backward).

Exercise 5.

The body is straight. The coccyx is leaned forward. The position of the lumbar spine is fixed. Keep your head straight. Fists are over the waist, they are in the kidney area. We try to bring the elbows together as close as possible. We make a few springy movements with our elbows towards each other in order to do this. The spine is tilted forward as if we stretch the bowstring from the occiput to the coccyx (elbows are the arrows).

Similarly, you have to do the exercise forward, but now our knees are slightly bent, and, arching the spine, we have to try to reach our knees with our nose.

The spine takes the form of a bow. Make sure that your loin is not tilted!

Exercise 6.

Legs are wider than shoulders, feet are "glued" to the floor and they are parallel to each other, hands on the shoulders, the pelvis and hips are fixed, and you have to look ahead.

Remove your eyes, then turn your head slowly and consistently, the shoulder girdle, chest and stomach are turned to the right. Twist the upper part of the spine from the shoulder to that point where there should be the waist theoretically.

We make a few springy movements in this position so that each next effort should lead to a slight increase of the angle of rotation. Check it: the pelvis, hips and feet should be fixed! You have to do it to the other side the same way.

I am putting you in remembrance: the spine is the axis of rotation.

## The lumbosacral spine.

As a result of this work on the spine the state of urogenital system improves, blood stasis in the pelvic organs is reduced, the pain, which is caused by the radiculitis, sciatica and other diseases, is removed, and sexuality is restored.

Attention!

If you have the hernias in the lumbosacral spine, all the exercises are done very carefully, with minimum amplitude!

Please, distribute the weight evenly throughout the spine.

Exercise 1.

The legs are half bent at the knees, hips are directed forward, and the upper part of the body is static.

We try to touch the top with the coccyx from the bottom, trying to reach the forehead with the pubis (not vice versa!), we alternate emerging tension with easy relaxation.

Do the exercise several times. Make sure that there are no tilts! The spine is bent backward in the form of an arc.

Exercise 2.

Tilt the tailbone and pelvis backward, legs are slightly bent at the knees, toes are slightly turned inwards, the upper part of the body is static. The head is straight!

Try to reach the back of the head with your coccyx. We make a few springy movements, alternating tension with relaxation. There are sensations in the lumbosacral area. You have to remove emerging heaviness by doing exercise? 1.

Exercise 3.

Knees can be slightly bent. The body is straight and is tilted forward at an angle of 45 °.

Trying to reach the occiput with your coccyx (not vice versa!), tilt your waist.

Don't throw your head back. Make 8-10 movements. Then, at this position, we transfer weight from one foot to the other repeatedly.

Remove the tension by doing exercise 1.


Exercise 4.

The knees are half bent; straight body is slightly tilted back. Head is straight!

We reach the back of the head with our coccyx. The butt is thrown back, the belly goes forward.

Look at your backbone with your inner eye. If you find a site where the tension is too strong, then we move power from there, evenly distributing it around the spinal column.

At this position, we go down lower and lower, alternately shifting the body weight from one leg to the other. Repeat this exercise several times. Remove the tension in the loin.

Exercise 5.

Make the circular movements of the hips at first 8-10 times in one direction and then the same number of movements in the other direction. The upper part of the body is static.

Exercise 6.

The body is straight, we move the hip to the right and forward, that is, body weight is transferred to the right. This is a starting position.

Make a few springy movements with the hip to the side, as if you push it further to the right.

Then, the initial position is fixed and the left side is stretched: left arm is raised vertically upward (at the worst, it is possible to put the palm on your occiput), the body is tilted to the right. Then, without changing the tilt, the body weight is transferred to the left leg and stretch the left side.

Similarly, do the exercises with the left hip and stretch the right side: try to touch the ceiling with your palm and make it easy to lean to the left.

Exercise 7.

Toes are slightly turned inward, the right hand is directed vertically upward, the left hand is put down. Try to touch the ceiling with your arm. Stretch your spine more and more and slightly bend your spine each time.

The same movements are repeated with the left hand.

Exercise 8.

Relax the whole body, massage the capillaries. Shake the muscles of the face, neck, arms, chest, abdomen, butt, hips and legs consistently.

Now do this exercise in reverse order. Imagine how a puppy does it, shaking off after a swim. And now you can relax and breathe as we did before the beginning of doing the complex of spine exercises.

## Twisting the spine.

Let me remind you: the spine is the axis of all movements. The head is in the line with the spine! The weight must be distributed evenly throughout the spine. Movements are flowing, don't allow painful sensations! Don't hold your breath!!!

### Exercise 1.

Feet are wider than shoulders, feet are "glued" to the floor and they are parallel to each other. Knees are slightly bent, hands are on the shoulder girdles.

Start with a smooth, slow, consistent body twist to failure to the right. There are eyes, head, shoulders, chest, abdomen, hips, pelvis, and legs – everything without feet. This is a starting position.

Then you have to make some effort to create tension, then you turn around further. Light relaxation and tension again, and so we do this exercise several times. Do a slow exhalation during each tension. Then return the starting position.

Attention!

When you feel pain, please, reduce the strain!

### Exercise 2.

Legs are wider than shoulders, feet are "glued" to the floor and they are parallel to each other, the body is tilted forward at an angle of 45 °, back is straight, hands are on the shoulder girdles.

Start the body rotation around a fixed spine to the right: the eyes, head, neck, shoulders, chest unfold to the ceiling, herewith your right elbow "looks" upward. Alternating tension with easy relaxation allows you to increase the angle of rotation gradually. After completing several of these alternations, return the starting position smoothly and slowly. You can straighten your body only after that! Do the same exercise to the right.

### Exercise 3.

Feet are wider than shoulders, feet are "glued" to the floor and they are parallel to each other. Back is straight, it is tilted backward, your head is in line with spine, and chin is pointed to his chest, your hands are on the shoulder girdles.

Exercise is similar to the previous one, but the leading elbow is pointed down when the body turns around, and your eyes look at the left heel over your shoulder. During twisting the spine down to the left side, you have to look at the right heel over your shoulder.

### Exercise 4.

Legs are wider than shoulders, feet are "glued" to the floor and they are parallel to each other. The body is tilted strongly to the right (tilts forward-backward are unacceptable!!!), back is straight.

The head is aligned with the spine.

The right elbow is a leading elbow and it moves backward and upward. The view is led away to the right; head, shoulders, chest turn around the axis of the spine and turn to the ceiling. Chin is put down.

Keep track of holding the tilt of your body to the right!

But that's not all!

Without changing the position of the body, spin the body to the left in reverse order.

At the same time the left elbow becomes the leading, it "goes" upward, backward and down, and the right elbow goes up, respectively. Look at the right heel over your left shoulder.

Make the reverse rotation of your body to the right in order to return the initial position.

Exercise 5.

You need to change the word "right" to "left" and vice versa everywhere in the description of previous twisting in order to do this exercise properly. Please, be careful and cautious.

If you still aren't sure that you are doing the exercise correctly, then take some expensive and fragile thing and do twisting near the wall, pressing and holding this thing with your head.

If the first attempt isn't successful, then an attempt is made as long as you learn it.

And these exercises can be done with a stick on your shoulders, but not under the whiplash!

Exercise 6.

Take a few quiet deep inhalations and exhalations, as we did it before doing the spine exercises.

# Complex of mandatory exercises.

I am putting you in remembrance that all these exercises are done without the glasses.

## Exercise «Stamp».

This exercise can be done both sitting and standing at the window. You have to decide for yourself how you will do it.

Glue a little mark or a picture, which size is 3 x 3 or 4 x 4 cm, on the glass, just below eye level. A picture must be cheerful, well-drawn, and green. Green is curative for the eyes. You have to look at live green as much as possible.

Select the object with the vague outlines from outside the window.

Attention!

During eye recovery the object is changed but we have to always choose it at a distance so that it couldn't be seen clearly. But you don't have to change the distance between the picture on the window and eyes (20-25 cm)!!!

And you begin to train the unit of accommodative apparatus of the eye. The duration of work is 10 minutes. Don't think about the time!

It is better to put light, relaxing, pleasant music.

We look at the drawing on the picture for 3-5 seconds, and then look at the selected object outside the window, and look at it over the mark which is glued to glass. Then look at the object for 3-5 seconds and look at the picture again.

Make sure to keep your eyes not popped out of head! If the tension appears, blink easily and flutter your eyelashes on the cheeks in order to relax the muscles!

This exercise should be done 2 times a day during daylight hours, but the time interval between sets should be at least two hours.

Are you okay? This is excellent! Keep it as long as possible!!!

# Do you know how to look at the sun?

People in the East have known how to treat any eye disease with the help of the sun since ancient times. But how did they do it?

1. It is useful to look at the sun with two eyes and let your tears fall, without blinking, but with strict adherence to certain rules.

You have to remember! It is possible to look at the sun with two eyes at sunrise or sunset, when the half of the disk is visible only at the line of the horizon, and this is particularly important! If the sun has already risen over the house or hasn't dropped half to the horizon yet, it is dangerous to look directly at it. It is dangerous to look at the sun, when it reaches its zenith!

You mustn't look at the sun motionlessly in no case, staring straight before one.

The exercise is done every day for one minute in the first week. The duration of doing exercise is gradually leaded up to two minutes during the second week. Later you have to increase the duration of exercise doing up to 10 minutes but not more than that.

All the birds live and die with perfect eyesight because they are the first to greet the dawn, and they don't look at the sun during the day. Everything is in harmony in nature.

2. Stand in the shade so that one half of your face is in shadow, and the other is in the sunlit area. Stand with your, feet which are wider than shoulder width, for stability.

Begin to turn your head so that the face is in the sun and in the shade.

The breathing is quiet. Turning the head to the left, you say mentally: "The sun is coming!" Turning the head to the right, you say mentally: "The sun is going down!" It is very important not to "cling to" the sun with your look, because you cannot "look" at the bright sun with your eyes and closed eyelids.

You have to increase the duration of doing the exercise up to 10 minutes gradually, starting with one minute.

After that, you have to do the exercise called "Relax". Relaxation is done at least two times longer than the exercise is done.

You have to alternate the exercises with long rest (the longer, the better).

3. Now we leave the shade and walk out into the sun. Exercise can be done during the day before 11 a.m. and after 3 p.m. You have to put your feet comfortably and start turning your body on the around the axis.

Don't you forget to take off your glasses? Eyes are closed. The head is raised slightly upwards, so that the sun is shining under your brows on your eyelids.

We make large turns of our body to the right, and we rive the left heel off the ground easily. The head follows the movements of the body.

Similarly, rive your right heel off the ground. Don't swing. This exercise should induce relaxation throughout the body.

During turning your body, say the phrase mentally: "The sun is passing me by to the left, then to the right, to the left again, and again and again, but all the time in the opposite direction of my turn"

Do you remember that we have explained why you need to think while doing exercises at the end of the previous exercise?

You have to relax again, do the exercise "Relax".

4. Stand on the sunlit land. Legs are put steadily. Cover one eye with your hand (it is still open). Head is tilted down. Going on turning your body, look at the ground around your legs, blinking as quickly as possible. Eye, which is covered with your hand, is blinking too.

Now look at the sun, and turn your body, while your eyes are blinking. One eye is still covered with your hand. Then, similarly, do this exercise with the other eye.

NB: if the sun reaches its zenith, you mustn't do this exercise!

# Breathing through eyes.

Before you start to do the exercise, read the description carefully,

Get on the image of youth!

Sit in a chair, make yourself comfortable. Hands are on knees, back is straight. All body and facial muscles are relaxed. There is peace in your body and soul. Breathe only through the nose. And now proceed.

Observe how you breathe through your nose. There is cold in your nose and nasopharynx when you inhale, there is warm when you exhale.

In any case, the inhaled air is cooler than the one that we exhale. You have to learn how to catch this slight fluctuation of temperature with your eyes.

Now imagine that you inhale and exhale through the nose, and your attention is on the eye area. Try to catch the air movement and temperature fluctuation with your eyes. You can do this exercise with open and closed eyes, do it as it is easier for you.

Such breathing gives excellent results, especially when you imagine that your eyes are healthy.

The eyes begin to see more clearly when you inhale, and with each exhalation veil leaves you, "flies" are disappearing, stress and fatigue are relieved, that is, everything that can be a cause of eye discomfort.

Now, you have to remember: the feeling of coolness (when you inhale) gives your eyes the best things, and a feeling of warmth (when you exhale) takes everything that prevents your eyes from being healthy. You can breathe through your eyes at anytime and anywhere. "Breathe" in order to be healthy!

Beware of doing the exercises reluctantly, as if by doing yourself a favor. You don't get any benefit and may even hurt yourself. Because thoughts are material!

## You reap what you sow!

This is morning! There is the ease and joy inside you because a new day has come, and you are open to new opportunities to make a lot of good things for yourself and others.

At first you will have to make great efforts to play the role of a happy and healthy person. Cultivate the habit of being happy and healthy. Every day you will be less and less in need for forcing yourself, because this role will become your inner essence gradually.

# Everything develops with training.

All exercises are done according to the "Meditation" with the Image of the youth. Merge with this Image together.

Every morning drink a glass of hot boiled water on an empty stomach. Imagine how this water passes through the cells and blood vessels of the whole body, purifying them and making them elastic.

Take a shower twice a day, in the morning and evening, and wash away the toxins and slags in order to prevent their reabsorption through the skin pores.

After morning exercises have a snack, don't be hungry. But you have to know when to stop, don't overeat. Otherwise it will be difficult to do the exercises.

## 1. Articular gymnastics.

Execution of the exercises will take about 35 minutes when you do it for the first time, for about a week. Once all the exercises have been mastered well, this time should not exceed 15-20 minutes. The main thing is to remember that you need to send 90% of your efforts to the artificial creation of the qualities through the creation of which you want to embody yourself. Doing mechanical exercises are a road to nowhere.

## 2. An exercise "Stamp". Do it twice a day for 10 minutes.

## 3. Eye exercises. You can do them several times during the day, it is very useful. But 1 time a day for 10 minutes is a must!

**4. Relaxation exercises called "Guiding energy to the eyes"; "Relax".** Do it as often as possible, but at least you have to do it for 10 minutes a day. Relaxation facilitates the faster recovery of vision and it is very useful for the entire nervous system.

**5. When you work with an eye chart, you correct your vision.** Do it twice a day, in the morning and after the afternoon.

Plan your work so that you have the opportunity to do eye exercises and relaxation before vision correction by using an eye chart ("Guiding energy to the eyes" and "Relax"). Don't forget to wash your hands! This is serious!

Do three sets three times for 30 seconds.

Hold the "muscle corset". Elate yourself; create the joyful expectation of the result in your soul artificially.

Do the first set for one and a half minutes, which is divided into 30 seconds. You have to work with both eyes. Then, do a relaxation exercise called "Relax"!

You have to increase your emotions as long as you don't notice the first glimpses of improvement of your sight in the table. Keep your spirits high!

A second approach. You have to turn around so that the light may fall on the table from a different angle and continue to exercise for 30 seconds. Similarly, then we have to repeat this exercise twice.

You have to give the relaxation to your eyes and entire nervous system again ("Relax").

Do the last set with each eye for 30 seconds alternately (the row for the exercise is selected for each of them according to the general scheme).

After that you have to do the "Relax"!

Do the exercise using your two eyes for the last 30 seconds.

Do relaxation exercises and create the sense of self-gratification in your soul at the end of the complex!!!

6. You have to work with the sun every morning for 10 minutes until 11 a.m.

7. Breathing through your eyes. Do it as often as possible. And you have to combine it with the exercise of the movement of sensations of heat, tingle and cold from the occiput to the eyeballs.

# Conclusion.

Work on the vision restoration can be distributed throughout the day by choosing a convenient time for practice, but following accident prevention, special conditions or other remarks. So, before you make an individual study plan, read again all the exercises carefully.

There is another piece of advice.

When you start to plan to work on yourself, various hindering circumstances appear very often.

You know that there are many intrigues of laziness. Trick it. Don't bind yourself to the time and training place.

Therefore, work on yourself permanently, change yourself, and the world around you will change too.

Four-six days are given to decrease the 1 dpt. You mustn't reduce the diopters faster because rapid and hard work can lead to inhibition of the recovery process. You also need to exercise for 1-3 days (depending on intensity) per week, apart from doing the exercises of "Meditation"!

You have obtained a huge flow of information and thus you have done considerable work on yourself. So, you are a different person! There are many ways, but you know that if you want to achieve something, you have to act!

The road is made by walking!

www.ingramcontent.com/pod-product-compliance
Lightning Source LLC
Chambersburg PA
CBHW062019280526
45787CB00005B/2166